more *Skinny*
SLOW COOKER
RECIPES
75 MORE DELICIOUS RECIPES UNDER 300, 400 AND 500 CALORIES

More Skinny Slow Cooker Recipes
75 More Delicious Recipes Under 300, 400 & 500 Calories From The No.1 Best Selling Amazon Author Of The Skinny Slow Cooker Recipe Book

A Bell & Mackenzie Publishing Limited Publication
First published in 2013 by Bell & Mackenzie Publishing
Limited
Copyright © Bell & Mackenzie Publishing Limited 2013

ISBN 978-1-909855-18-2

A CIP catalogue record of this book is available from the
British Library

Disclaimer
The information and advice in this book is intended as
a guide only. If using the recipes as part of a diet, any
individual should independently seek the advice of a
doctor or health professional before embarking on any
diet or weight loss plan. We do not recommend a calorie
controlled diet if you are pregnant, breastfeeding, elderly
or under 18 years of age. Some recipes may contain nuts or
traces of nuts. Those suffering from any allergies associated
with nuts should avoid any recipes containing nuts or nut
based oils.avoid any recipes containing nuts or nut based
oils.

Contents

Contents

Contents

Introduction

Welcome to **More Skinny Slow Cooker Recipes**: 75 More Delicious Recipes Under 300, 400 & 500 Calories From The No.1 Best Selling Amazon Author of *The Skinny Slow Cooker Recipe Book.*

This new collection of recipes compliments the hugely successful 'The Skinny Slow Cooker Recipe Book' also by CookNation, which became a No.1 Amazon best seller with its collection of skinny, low calorie slow cooker dishes for those wishing to maintain a balanced, healthy diet. Its popularity prompted this new collection of recipes with fresh inspiration to prepare more tasty recipes all falling under 300, 400 or 500 calories.

If you haven't already, you can find the original 'The Skinny Slow Cooker Recipe Book' on Amazon.

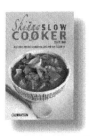

The slow cooker allows you to prepare delicious meals with the minimum of preparation and fuss. With as little as just 15 minutes prep you can have a low calorie, nutritious and tasty meal slowly cooking whilst you get on with the things you need to do. If you have a family to cook for, a busy life that means you start early and are out for most of the day, or just don't want to be tied to the kitchen for hours, then the slow cooker is your saviour. Slow cooking enables you to get on with other things without worrying that your food will overcook, spill-over or burn. The slow cooking process brings out all the best flavours of your ingredients without losing out on goodness. It's easy to use, delivers great results and with our skinny slow cooking recipes you can be confident you are preparing low calorie, healthy dishes as part of a wholesome diet.

If you have already read one of the other 'Skinny' titles from CookNation you may be familiar with some of the following information, in which case please feel free to skip straight to our recipes. If however your slow cooker has been stored in a cupboard over the summer months or you have just purchased a slow cooker for the first time, we recommend reading the following pages to familiarise yourself with how to get the best out of your appliance and advice on using our recipes.

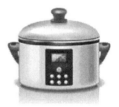 During the colder months our bodies naturally crave warm, filling and comforting food, which can often result in overeating, weight gain and sluggishness.

These delicious recipes use simple and inexpensive fresh and store-cupboard ingredients, are packed full of flavour and goodness, and show that you can enjoy maximum taste with minimum calories.

Each recipe has been tried, tested, and enjoyed time and time again and, with 75 new delicious recipes to choose from, we're sure you'll soon agree that diet can still mean delicious!

Preparation
- All the recipes should take no longer than 10-15 minutes to prepare. Browning the meat will make a difference to the

taste of your recipe, but if you really don't have the time, don't worry - it will still taste great.
- All meat and vegetables should be cut into even sized pieces unless stated in the recipes. Some ingredients can take longer to cook than others, particularly root vegetables, but that has been allowed for in the cooking time.
- As much as possible meat should be trimmed of visible fat and the skin removed.

Low Cost

Slow cooking is ideal for cheaper meat cuts. The 'tougher' cuts used in this collection of recipes are transformed into meat which melts-in-your-mouth and helps to keep costs down. We've also made sure not to include one-off ingredients which are used for a single recipe and never used again. All the herbs and spices listed can be used in multiple recipes throughout the book.

Slow Cooker Tips

- All cooking times are a guide. Make sure you get to know your own slow cooker so that you can adjust timings accordingly.
- Read the manufacturers operating instructions as appliances can vary. For example, some recommend preheating the slow cooker for 20 minutes before use whilst others advocate switching on only when you are ready to start cooking.
- Slow cookers do not brown-off meat. While this is not always necessary, if you do prefer to brown your meat you must first do this in a pan with a little low calorie cooking spray.
- A spray of one calorie cooking oil in the cooker before

adding ingredients will help with cleaning or you can buy liners.

• Don't be tempted to regularly lift the lid of your appliance while cooking. The seal that is made with the lid on is all part of the slow cooking process. Each time you do lift the lid you will need to increase the cooking time.

• Removing the lid at the end of the cooking time can be useful to thicken up a sauce by adding additional cooking time and continuing to cook without the lid on. On the other hand if perhaps a sauce it too thick removing the lid and adding a little more liquid can help.

• Always add hot liquids to your slow cooker, not cold.

• Do not overfill your slow cooker.

• Allow the inner dish of your slow cooker to completely cool before cleaning. Any stubborn marks can usually be removed after a period of soaking in hot soapy water.

• Be confident with your cooking. Feel free to use substitutes to suit your own taste and don't let a missing herb or spice stop you making a meal - you'll almost always be able to find something to replace it.

Our Recipes

 The recipes in this book are all low calorie dishes mainly serving 4, which makes it easier for you to monitor your overall daily calorie intake as well as those you are cooking for. The recommended daily calories are approximately 2000 for women and 2500 for men.

Broadly speaking, by consuming the recommended levels of calories each day you should maintain your current weight. Reducing the number of calories (a calorie deficit) will result in losing weight. This happens because the body begins to use fat stores for energy to make up the reduction in calories, which in turn results in weight loss. We have already counted the calories for each dish making it easy for you to fit this into your daily eating plan whether you want to lose weight, maintain your current figure or are just looking for some great-tasting, skinny slow cooker meals.

I'm Already On A Diet. Can I Use These Recipes?

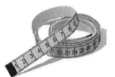 Yes of course. All the recipes can be great accompaniments to many of the popular calorie-counting diets. We all know that sometimes dieting can result in hunger pangs, cravings and boredom from eating the same old foods day in and day out. Our skinny slow cooker recipes provide filling meals that should satisfy you for hours afterwards.

I Am Only Cooking For One. Will This Book Work For Me?

Yes. We would recommend following the method for 4 servings then dividing and storing the rest in single size portions for you to use in the future. Most of the recipes will freeze well. Allow your slow cooked meals to cool to room temperature before refrigerating or freezing. When ready to defrost, allow to thaw in a fridge overnight then at room temperature for a few hours depending on the size of portion. Reheat thoroughly.

Nutrition

All of the recipes in this collection are balanced low calorie meals that should keep you feeling full and help you avoid snacking in-between meals.

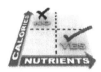

If you are following a diet, it is important to balance your food between proteins, good carbs, dairy, fruit and vegetables.

11

Protein
Keeps you feeling full and is also essential for building body tissue. Good protein sources come from meat, fish and eggs.

Carbohydrates
Carbs are generally high in calories, which makes them difficult to include in a calorie limiting diet. Carbs are a good source of energy for your body as they are converted more easily into glucose (sugar), providing energy. Try to eat 'good carbs' which are high in fibre and nutrients e.g. whole fruits and veg, nuts, seeds, whole grain cereals, beans and legumes.

Dairy
Dairy products provide you with vitamins and minerals. Cheeses can be high in calories but other products such as fat free Greek yoghurt, crème fraiche and skimmed milk are all good.

Fruit & Vegetables
Eat your five a day. There is never a better time to fill your 5 a day quota. Not only are fruit and veg very healthy, they also fill up your plate and are ideal snacks when you are feeling hungry.

We have adopted the broader nutritional principals in all our recipes.

Portion Sizes
The majority of recipes are for 4 servings. The calorie count is based on one serving.

It is important to remember that if you are aiming to lose

weight using any of our skinny recipes, the size of the portion that you put on your plate will significantly affect your weight loss efforts. Filling your plate with over-sized portions will obviously increase your calorie intake and hamper your dieting efforts.

It is important with all meals that you use a correct sized portion, which generally is the size of your clenched fist. This applies to any side dishes of vegetables and carbs too.

Calorie Conscious Side Suggestions

If you want to make any of the recipes in this book more bulky, you may want to add a further accompaniment to them. Here's a list of some key side vegetables, salad, noodles etc that you may find useful when working out your calories.

All calories are per 100g/3 ½ oz. Rice and noodle measurements are cooked weights.

Asparagus:	20 cals
Beansprouts:	30 cals
Brussel Sprouts:	42 cals
Butternut Squash:	45 cals
Cabbage:	30 cals
Carrots:	41 cals
Cauliflower:	25 cals
Celery:	14 cals
Courgette/zucchini:	16 cals
Cucumber:	15 cals
Egg noodles:	62 cals
Green beans:	81 cals
Leeks:	61 cals
Long grain rice:	140 cals
Mixed salad leaves:	17 cals

Mixed salad leaves:	30 cals
Mushrooms:	22 cals
Pak choi:	13 cals
Parsnips:	67 cals
Peas:	64 cals
Pepper (bell):	20 cals
Potatoes:	75 cals
Rocket:	17 cals
Spinach:	23 cals
Sweet Potato:	86 cals
Sweet corn:	86 cals
Tomatoes:	18 cals

All Recipes Are A Guide Only

All the recipes in this book are a guide only. You may need to alter quantities and cooking times to suit your own appliances.

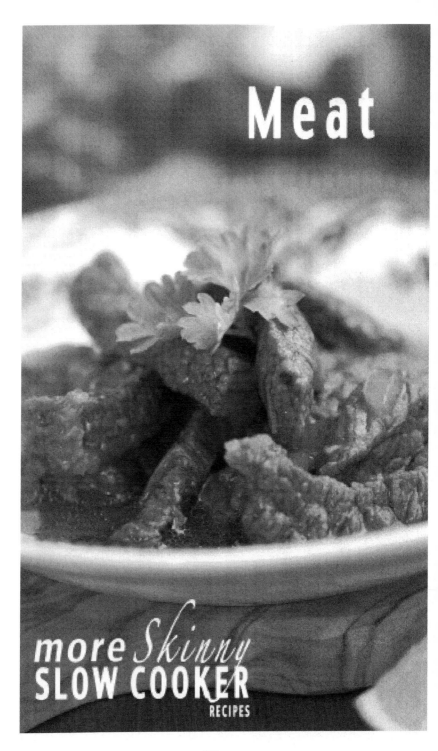

Meat

more *Skinny*
SLOW COOKER
RECIPES

Melting Beef Topside & Spinach
Serves 4

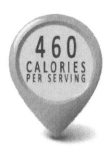

460 CALORIES PER SERVING

Ingredients:

1kg/2¼lb piece lean beef topside
3 carrots, chopped
2 onions, chopped
2 parsnips, chopped
1 celery stalk, chopped
1 tbsp olive oil
1 tsp each ground coriander/cilantro, thyme & salt
½ tsp ground cinnamon
500ml/2 cups chicken stock/broth
400g/14oz spinach
1 large bunch freshly chopped flat leaf parsley
Salt & pepper to taste

Method:

• Trim the beef of any visible fat and season well with salt & pepper.
• Gently sauté the carrots, onions, parsnips and celery in the olive oil for a few minutes until softened.
• Add the coriander, thyme, salt & cinnamon and stir well. Put the sautéed vegetables, beef and stock into the slow cooker.
• Cover and leave to cook on low for 8-10 hours or until the beef is meltingly tender.
• Add the spinach to the slow cooker and cook for 10-20 minutes or until the spinach gently wilts.
• Remove the beef from the slow cooker. Slice thinly and arrange on plates with the chopped vegetables and wilted spinach.
• Sprinkle with chopped parsley and serve.

You could try substituting half the chicken stock for white wine if you prefer but be aware this will increase the calories of the dish.

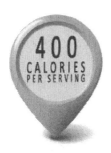

400
CALORIES
PER SERVING

Moroccan Beef
& Sweet Potatoes
Serves 4

Method:

- Trim the beef of any visible fat and season well with salt & pepper.
- Peel the sweet potatoes and slice thinly.
- Gently sauté the carrots & onions in the olive oil for a few minutes until softened.
- Add the turmeric, cumin, coriander, cayenne pepper & paprika and stir.
- Put the sautéed vegetables, beef and stock into the slow cooker. Arrange the sliced sweet potatoes over the top. Cover and leave to cook on high for 5-7 hours or until the beef & sweet potatoes are tender.
- Adjust the seasoning, sprinkle with chopped parsley and serve.

Adjust the cayenne pepper in this dish if you prefer it a little spicier.

Ingredients:

500g/1lb 2oz lean stewing steak, cubed
450g/1lb sweet potatoes
2 carrots, chopped
1 onion, sliced
1 tbsp olive oil
½ tsp each turmeric, cumin, coriander/cilantro, cayenne pepper & paprika
250ml/1 cup beef stock/ broth
1 small bunch freshly chopped flat leaf parsley
Salt & pepper to taste

17

Lentil Beef Meatballs & Rice
Serves 4

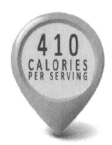

410 CALORIES PER SERVING

Ingredients:

250g/9oz lean minced/
ground beef
200g/7oz red lentils
1 free range egg
1 garlic clove, crushed
2 tbsp freshly chopped flat
leaf parsley
1 onion, finely chopped
400g/14oz tinned chopped
tomatoes
½ tsp brown sugar
2 tbsp tomato puree/paste
2 tbsp worcestershire
sauce
200g/7oz long grain rice
Salt & pepper to taste

Method:

• Combine the beef, lentils, egg, garlic, parsley and onion together in a bowl.
• Use your hands to shape into small meatballs (about half the size of a table tennis ball).
• Add the meatballs to the slow cooker along with the chopped tomatoes, sugar, tomato puree & worcestershire sauce.
• Cover and leave to cook on low for 5-6 hours or until the meatballs are cooked through.
• Meanwhile cook the rice in salted boiling water until tender.
• Place the drained rice in shallow bowls and spoon the meatballs and sauce over the top.
• Season and serve.

Add a little beef stock to the slow cooker if you feel the sauce is drying out too much during cooking.

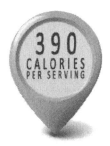

390 CALORIES PER SERVING

Garlic & Lamb Stew
Serves 4

Method:

- Heat the olive oil in a pan. Season the lamb and brown in the hot oil for a few minutes.
- Remove from the pan and place in a small plastic bag with the flour. Shake well to cover each piece of lamb in flour.
- Place the floured lamb in the slow cooker along with the onions, garlic, paprika, cumin, stock, broad beans & spinach.
- Cover and leave to cook on high for 4-6 hours or until the lamb is tender and cooked through.
- Season and serve.

Ingredients:

500g/1lb 2oz lamb fillet, cubed
1 tbsp olive oil
1 tbsp plain/all purpose flour
1 onion, finely chopped
4 cloves garlic, crushed
1 tsp paprika
½ tsp cumin
250ml/1 cup chicken stock/broth
300g/11oz broad beans
200g/7oz spinach
Salt & pepper to taste

Shelled, fresh or frozen broad beans will work fine. If you prefer your vegetables crunchy add the beans and spinach towards the end of the cooking time.

Cider Pork & Beans
Serves 4

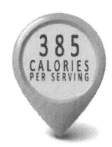

385 CALORIES PER SERVING

Ingredients:

450g/1lb pork tenderloin, cubed
1 tbsp plain/all purpose flour
1 onion, finely chopped
2 cloves garlic, crushed
2 celery stalks, chopped
1 tbsp dried thyme
75g/3oz frozen peas
400g/14oz tinned flageolet beans, drained
250ml/1 cup dry cider
Salt & pepper to taste

Method:

• Season the pork pieces and place in a small plastic bag with the flour.
• Shake well to cover each piece of meat. Place the floured pork in the slow cooker along with all the other ingredients.
• Cover and leave to cook on high for 4-6 hours or until the pork is tender and cooked through.
• Season and serve.

Add a little more cider or chicken stock to the slow cooker if you feel the sauce needs it.

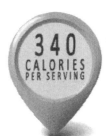

340
CALORIES
PER SERVING

Pork Tenderloin With Sage & Orange

Serves 4

Method:

- Season the pork and spray with a little low cal cooking oil.
- Heat a frying pan and evenly brown the pork for a minute or two. Place the meat in the slow cooker.
- Grate the zest off the orange and juice the flesh. Add the orange zest and juice to the slow cooker along with the onion, garlic, sage leaves, broccoli and chicken stock.
- Cover and leave to cook on high for 4-6 hours or until the pork is tender and cooked through.
- Take the pork out of the cooker and slice thickly.
- Arrange on plates, add the broccoli to the side and spoon over the orange sauce.

Ingredients:

500g/1lb 2oz pork tenderloin piece
1 orange
1 onion, finely chopped
2 cloves garlic, crushed
1 tbsp freshly chopped sage leaves
400g/14oz tenderstem broccoli spears
250ml/1 cup chicken stock/broth
Low cal cooking oil spray
Salt & pepper to taste

If you wanted a thicker sauce you could mix a little cornflour with warm water and add to the slow cooker.

Black Eyed Bean & Sausage Casserole
Serves 4

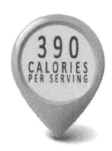

390 CALORIES PER SERVING

Ingredients:

150g/5oz lean back bacon, chopped

200g/7oz lean pork sausages

200g/7oz tinned black-eyed beans, drained

3 carrots, chopped

1 onion, chopped

3 cloves garlic, crushed

200g/7oz shredded greens

120ml/½ cup chicken stock/broth

Low cal cooking oil spray

Salt & pepper to taste

Method:

• Heat a frying pan and evenly brown the sausages and bacon for a minute or two in a little low cal cooking oil.

• Remove from the pan and slice the sausages with a sharp knife into thick 2cm/1inch discs.

• Add to the slow cooker along with all the other ingredients.

• Cover and leave to cook on high for 3-4 hours or until the sausages are cooked through and the vegetables are tender.

Bags of shredded greens are readily available in most supermarkets but are also easy enough to chop up and prepare yourself.

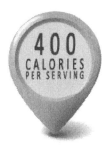

400 CALORIES PER SERVING

Paprika Pork Goulash
Serves 4

Method:

- Season the pork tenderloin.
- Gently sauté the peppers, onions & garlic in a little low cal spray for a few minutes until softened.
- Add all the ingredients, except the rice and yoghurt, to the slow cooker.
- Cover and leave to cook on high for 4-6 hours or until the pork is cooked through.
- At the end of the cooking time stir the yoghurt through.
- Meanwhile cook the rice in salted boiling water until tender.
- Drain and serve as a bed for the pork.

Ingredients:

**500g/1lb 2oz pork tenderloin, cubed
2 red (bell) peppers, sliced
1 onion, sliced
2 garlic cloves, crushed
2 tbsp paprika
½ tsp cayenne pepper
250ml/1 cup tomato passata/sieved tomatoes
½ tsp each salt & brown sugar
60ml/¼cup chicken stock/broth
200g/7oz long grain rice
2 tbsp fat free Greek yoghurt
Low cal cooking oil spray
Salt & pepper to taste**

Paprika is a lovely gently 'warming' spice, whilst the cayenne pepper adds the 'kick'.

Pork & Garlic Curry
Serves 4

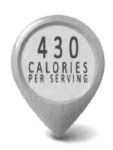

Ingredients:

**500g/1lb 2oz pork
tenderloin, cubed
1 green (bell) pepper, very
finely sliced
1 onion, finely sliced
5 garlic cloves, crushed
1 tbsp freshly grated
ginger
2 tbsp fish sauce
1 tsp each turmeric &
brown sugar
1 tbsp Thai red curry paste
120ml/½ cup tomato
passata/sieved tomatoes
60ml/¼ cup chicken stock/
broth
½ tsp each salt & brown
sugar
60ml/¼ cup low fat
coconut milk
200g/7oz basmati rice
Low cal cooking oil spray
Salt & pepper to taste**

Method:

• Season the pork tenderloin.
• Gently sauté the peppers, onions, garlic & ginger in a little low cal spray for a few minutes until softened.
• Add all the ingredients, except the coconut milk & rice, to the slow cooker. Cover and leave to cook on high for 4-6 hours or until the pork is cooked through and tender.
• At the end of the cooking time stir the coconut milk through.
• Meanwhile cook the rice in salted boiling water until tender.
• Drain, season and serve with the curry.

This curry packs a lot of flavour with its blend of Thai paste, coconut milk, garlic and fish sauce.

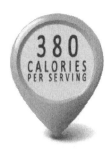

380
CALORIES
PER SERVING

Fontina Cheese Omelette
Serves 4

Method:

• Place the onions and potatoes in a food processor and whizz until finely chopped.

• Season well and gently sauté in the olive oil for a few minutes until softened.

• Break the eggs into a cup and whisk. Combine the sautéed potatoes and onions in a bowl with the eggs, cheese, chorizo & parsley.

• Add to the slow cooker, cover and leave to cook on high for 1-2 hours or until the eggs are set and the omelette is piping hot.

• Serve in wedges with the shredded lettuce.

Ingredients:

2 onions, finely sliced
300g/11oz potatoes
1 tbsp olive oil
8 free range eggs
125g/4oz fontina cheese, chopped
125g/4oz chorizo sausage
4 tbsp freshly grated flat leaf parsley
2 romaine lettuces, shredded
Salt & pepper to taste

You may find it easier to add a liner to the slow cooker before you begin cooking so you can lift the entire omelette out whole. If you can't source fontina cheese you could substitute for gruyere.

Chorizo & Cabbage Hash
Serves 4

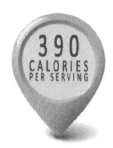

390 CALORIES PER SERVING

Ingredients:

2 onions, finely sliced
500g/1lb 2oz potatoes, cubed
1 tbsp olive oil
60ml/¼ cup chicken stock/ broth
1 pointed cabbage, shredded
200g/7oz chorizo sausage, chopped
Salt & pepper to taste

Method:

• Place all the ingredients in the slow cooker.
• Combine well, cover and leave to cook on high for 3-4 hours or until the potatoes are tender.
• Serve with lots of black pepper.

You could add some anchovy fillets to this dish to give it a deeper, salty depth.

26

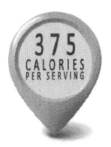

375
CALORIES
PER SERVING

Ham, Peppers & Eggs
Serves 4

Method:

- Place all the ingredients, except the eggs, in the slow cooker.
- Combine well, cover and leave to cook on high for 2-3 hours.
- After this time make 4 'wells' in the slow cooker. Crack the eggs into these wells.
- Season and leave to cook until the eggs are set.

Ingredients:

2 onions, finely sliced
2 garlic cloves, crushed
2 red (bell) peppers, sliced
200g/7oz cooked lean ham, chopped
200g/7oz courgettes/ zucchini, sliced lengthways
1 tsp paprika
1 tbsp tomato puree/paste
50g/2oz sundried tomatoes, chopped
400g/14oz tinned chopped tomatoes
75g/3oz low fat cheddar cheese, grated
4 tbsp freshly grated flat leaf parsley
4 free range eggs
Salt & pepper to taste

Chopped coriander will also work well in this dish.

27

Rump Steak &
Mixed Mushrooms
Serves 4

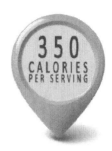

350 CALORIES PER SERVING

Ingredients:

500g/1lb 2oz rump streak, thickly sliced
1 tbsp freshly grated ginger
2 garlic cloves, crushed
1 carrot, cut into fine matchsticks
2 onions, finely sliced
1 tbsp fish sauce
300g/11oz mixed mushrooms, sliced
1 chilli, deseeded and finely sliced
120ml/½ cup chicken stock/broth
½ tsp brown sugar
1 bunch spring onions/ scallions, finely sliced lengthways
2 tbsp soy sauce
200g/7oz fine egg noodles
Salt & pepper to taste

Method:

• Place all the ingredients, except the noodles, in the slow cooker.
• Combine well, cover and leave to cook on low for 4-6 hours or until the steak is tender.
• Meanwhile cook the noodles in salted boiling water until tender.
• Drain and serve with the steak & mushrooms.

Use any combination of mushrooms you like for this recipe. Shitake & oyster mushrooms work particularly well.

28

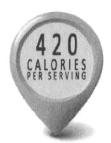

420
CALORIES
PER SERVING

Best Beef Tacos
Serves 4

Method:

- Place all the ingredients, except the taco shells, yoghurt & lettuce, in the slow cooker.
- Combine well, cover and leave to cook on high for 4-6 hours or until the mince is tender and cooked through.
- Serve the mince in taco shells with yoghurt and shredded lettuce on the top.

Ingredients:

500g/1lb 2oz lean minced/ ground beef
1 garlic clove, crushed
2 onions, sliced
1 tsp each cumin, paprika & cayenne pepper
½ tsp ground ginger
1 red (bell) pepper, finely chopped
2 tbsp worcestershire sauce
2 tbsp tomato puree/paste
400g/14oz tinned chopped tomatoes
8 Old El Paso taco shells
4 tbsp fat free Greek yoghurt
2 romaine lettuces, shredded
Salt & pepper to taste

Grated cheese is good on tacos too but it will increase the calorie count - so don't overdo it!

Highland Venison Stew

Serves 4

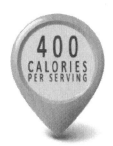

400 CALORIES PER SERVING

Ingredients:

500g/1lb 2oz venison
stewing steak, cubed
1 tbsp plain/all purpose
flour
½ tsp ground all spice
2 carrots, chopped
1 garlic clove, crushed
1 onion, sliced
2 celery stalks, sliced
380ml/1½ cups chicken
stock/broth
2 tbsp worcestershire
sauce
300g/11oz tenderstem
broccoli spears
300g/11oz new potatoes,
sliced
Low cal cooking oil spray
Salt & pepper to taste

Method:

• Season the venison and brown in a hot frying pan with a little low cal oil for a few minutes.
• Remove from the pan and place in a small plastic bag with the flour and all spice. Shake well to cover each piece of venison in flour.
• Place the floured meat in the slow cooker along with all the other ingredients.
• Cover and leave to cook on high for 4-6 hours or until the venison is tender and cooked through.
• Season and serve.

Venison is a tasty, low fat game meat which is now readily available in most supermarkets.

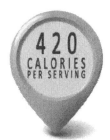

Beef & Stout Stew

Serves 4

Method:

- Season the beef and brown in a hot frying pan with a little low cal oil for a few minutes.
- Remove from the pan and place in a small plastic bag with the flour. Shake well to cover each piece of beef in flour.
- Place the floured meat in the slow cooker along with all the other ingredients.
- Cover and leave to cook on high for 4-6 hours or until the beef is tender and cooked through.
- Season and serve.

Ingredients:

500g/1lb 2oz beef stewing steak, cubed
1 tbsp plain/all purpose flour
2 carrots, sliced
1 parsnip, sliced
2 garlic cloves, crushed
1 onion, sliced
2 celery stalks, sliced
380ml/1½ cups stout beer
1 tsp English mustard
2 tbsp tomato puree/paste
300g/11oz spinach
300g/11oz new potatoes, sliced
Low cal cooking oil spray
Salt & pepper to taste

Guinness is good but you can use any type of good quality stout beer you prefer.

Pancetta & Beef Hot Pot
Serves 4

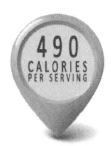

490
CALORIES
PER SERVING

Ingredients:

400g/1lb beef stewing steak, cubed
1 tbsp plain/all purpose flour
200g/7oz pancetta/Italian bacon, cubed
1 onion, sliced
2 carrots, sliced
1 parsnip, sliced
2 garlic cloves, crushed
2 celery stalks, sliced
60ml/¼ cup chicken stock/ broth
1 tsp marmite
2 tbsp tomato puree/paste
200g/7oz tinned chopped tomatoes
400g/11oz potatoes, sliced
Low cal cooking oil spray
Salt & pepper to taste

Method:

• Season the beef and place in a small plastic bag with the flour. Shake well to cover each piece of beef in flour.
• Gently sauté the pancetta and onions in a little low cal spray for a few minutes until the onions are golden.
• Place the floured meat in the slow cooker along with all the other ingredients - finishing with the sliced potatoes layered on top.
• Cover and leave to cook on high for 4-6 hours or until both the beef and potatoes are tender.
• Season and serve.

You could substitute the marmite for anchovy sauce instead.

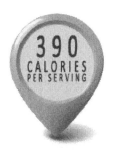

Coriander & Five Spice Pork
Serves 4

Method:

- Place all the ingredients, except the rice, in the slow cooker.
- Combine well, cover and leave to cook on high for 4-6 hours or until the pork is cooked through.
- Meanwhile cook the rice in salted boiling water until tender.
- Drain and serve with the spiced pork.

Reserve a little of the chopped coriander for garnish.

Ingredients:

500g/1lb 2oz pork tenderloin, cubed
1 red (bell) pepper, sliced
1 onion, sliced
2 celery stalks
2 garlic cloves, crushed
200ml/7oz vine ripened tomatoes, chopped
120ml/½ cup chicken stock/broth
2 tbsp tomato puree/paste
1 tsp Chinese 5 spice powder
1 large bunch freshly chopped coriander/ cilantro
200g/7oz long grain rice
Salt & pepper to taste

Beef & Beetroot
Serves 4

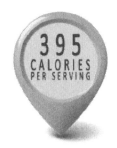

395 CALORIES PER SERVING

Ingredients:

500g/1lb 2oz stewing steak, cubed
300g/11oz beetroot, peeled & diced
1 onion, sliced
2 celery stalks
2 garlic cloves, crushed
3 bay leaves
200ml/7oz vine ripened tomatoes, chopped
120ml/½ cup beef stock/broth
1 tbsp tomato puree/paste
1 tbsp balsamic vinegar
4 tbsp freshly chopped flat leaf parsley
200g/7oz long grain rice
Low cal cooking oil spray
Salt & pepper to taste

Method:

• Place all the ingredients, except the rice, in the slow cooker.
• Combine well, cover and leave to cook on high for 4-6 hours or until the steak is soft and cooked through.
• Meanwhile cook the rice in salted boiling water until tender.
• Drain and serve with the stew.

You could add a little red wine in place of some beef stock if you like.

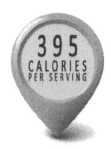

395 CALORIES PER SERVING

Pork & Sweetcorn With Couscous
Serves 4

Method:

• Place all the ingredients, except the couscous and stock cube, in the slow cooker.

• Combine well, cover and leave to cook on high for 4-6 hours or until the pork is tender.

• Meanwhile place the stock cube in boiling water and add the couscous.

• Cook until tender and drain if necessary.

• Fluff the couscous up with a fork and serve with the pork & sweetcorn stew.

Ingredients:

500g/1lb 2oz pork tenderloin, cubed
200g/7oz sweetcorn
2 onions, sliced
2 celery stalks
2 garlic cloves, crushed
1 tbsp dried oregano
1 tsp brown sugar
200g/7oz cherry tomatoes, halved
120ml/½ cup chicken stock/broth
1 tsp each ground cumin & coriander/cilantro
200g/7oz couscous
1 chicken stock cube
Salt & pepper to taste

Frozen sweetcorn is fine to use with this recipe but fresh kernels are great too.

35

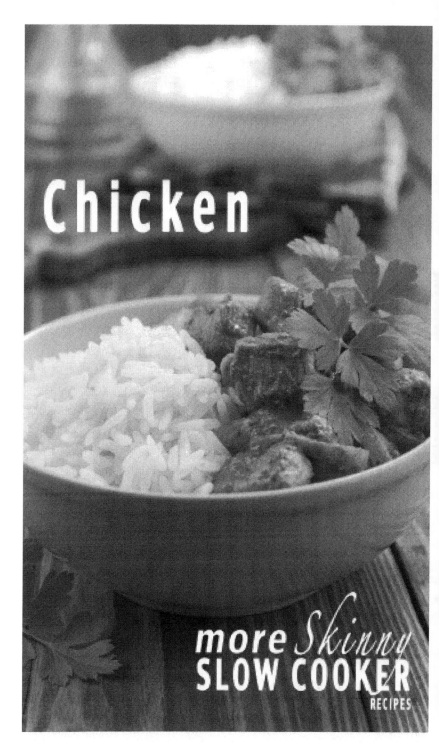

Chicken

more *Skinny*
SLOW COOKER
RECIPES

Red Wine Chicken & Grapes
Serves 4

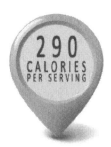

290 CALORIES PER SERVING

Ingredients:

4 x skinless chicken breasts each weighing 125g/4oz
120ml/½ cup red wine
120ml/½ cup chicken stock/broth
1 tbsp red pesto
2 red onions, sliced
125g/4oz red seedless grapes, halved
4 tbsp freshly chopped basil
200g/7oz watercress
Salt & pepper to taste

Method:

• Season the chicken breasts.
• Mix the red wine, stock and pesto together.
• Add all the ingredients, except the basil & watercress, to the slow cooker. Cover and leave to cook on high for 3-4 hours or until the chicken breasts are cooked through.
• Place the chicken breasts on plates and spoon over the sauce, grapes and onions.
• Add the watercress to the side of each plate, sprinkle the chicken with fresh basil and serve.

If you want to make this alcohol-free and reduce the calories, leave out the wine and double the chicken stock quantity.

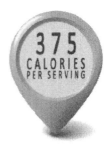

375 CALORIES PER SERVING

Method:

- Season the chicken breasts.
- Mix the cornflour with a little warm water to make a paste. Whisk the paste together with the lemon juice, lime cordial, sugar & salt.
- Add all the ingredients, except the spring onions and noodles, to the slow cooker. Cover and leave to cook on high for 3-4 hours or until the chicken breasts are cooked through.
- Meanwhile cook the noodles in salted boiling water until tender.
- Cut the chicken breasts diagonally into thick slices.
- Place the drained noodles in a shallow bowl, add the chicken slices and spoon the lemon sauce and vegetables over the top.
- Sprinkle with chopped spring onions and serve.

Add a little more water to the slow cooker during cooking if the sauce is thickening too much.

Ingredients:

4 x skinless chicken breasts each weighing 125g/4oz
2 tsp cornflour
4 tbsp lemon juice
3 tbsp lime cordial
2 tbsp brown sugar
½ tsp salt
180ml/¾ cup chicken stock/broth
1 onion, sliced
75g/3oz green beans, chopped
2 carrots, cut into thin batons
1 bunch spring onions/ scallions, chopped
200g/7oz fine egg noodles
Salt & pepper to taste

Spiced Eastern Chicken
Serves 4

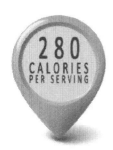

280 CALORIES PER SERVING

Ingredients:

**4 x skinless chicken breasts
each weighing 125g/4oz
½ tsp each ground
coriander/cilantro,
turmeric, cumin, nutmeg
& ginger
Pinch of salt & brown
sugar
120ml/½ cup chicken
stock/broth
1 onion, sliced
1 carrot, cut into
matchsticks
4 tbsp fat free Greek
yoghurt
1 tsp paprika
200g/7oz watercress
Salt & pepper to taste**

Method:

• Season the chicken breasts.
• Add all the ingredients, except the yoghurt, paprika & watercress, to the slow cooker. Combine well, cover and leave to cook on high for 3-4 hours or until the chicken breasts are cooked through.
• Cut the chicken breasts diagonally into thick slices and serve on a bed of watercress.
• Put 1 tbsp of yoghurt onto each plate. Sprinkle the yoghurt with paprika and serve.

This recipe is suitable for all the family but you could double the spice quantities if you prefer a particularly powerful dish.

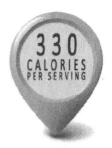

330
CALORIES
PER SERVING

Fennel & Garlic
Chicken
Serves 4

Method:

- Season the chicken breasts.
- Gently sauté the leeks, chopped fennel and garlic in a little low cal spray for a few minutes.
- Add all the ingredients, except the spinach & parsley, to the slow cooker. Combine well, cover and leave to cook on high for 3-4 hours or until the chicken breasts are cooked through.
- A few minutes before the cooking time is over add the spinach to the slow cooker to gently wilt.
- Cut the chicken breasts diagonally into thick slices and serve sprinkled with chopped parsley.

Ingredients:

4 x skinless chicken breasts each weighing 125g/4oz
2 leeks, sliced
1 fennel bulb, chopped
3 garlic cloves, crushed
400g/14oz tinned butter beans, rinsed
250ml/1 cup chicken stock/broth
125g/4oz spinach, chopped
4 tbsp freshly chopped flat leaf parsley
Low cal cooking oil spray
Salt & pepper to taste

You could add a little more stock or some dry white wine during cooking if the dish needs more liquid.

41

Root Veg & Chicken Pasta
Serves 4

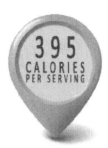

395 CALORIES PER SERVING

Ingredients:

400g/14oz skinless chicken breasts, sliced
2 onions, chopped
1 carrot, finely chopped
½ celeriac, finely chopped
1 parsnip, finely chopped
1 sweet potato, finely chopped
1 garlic clove, crushed
75g/3oz green beans, roughly chopped
370ml/1½ cups chicken stock/broth
4 tbsp freshly chopped flat leaf parsley
200g/7oz orzo pasta
Salt & pepper to taste

Method:

• Add all the ingredients, except the orzo pasta, to the slow cooker.
• Combine well, cover and leave to cook on high for 3-4 hours or until the chicken is cooked through and the vegetables are tender.
• Half an hour before the cooking time is over add the pasta.
• Combine really well and cook until tender.
• Season and serve.

You can use whichever small pasta shapes you prefer for this dish. Plenty of liquid is needed for the pasta to cook in, if there isn't enough, add a little more stock when you add the pasta.

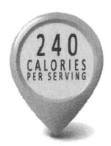

240 CALORIES PER SERVING

Olives, Chicken & Lemons

Serves 4

Method:

- Season the chicken breasts.
- Rub the turmeric and cinnamon into each one.
- Add all the ingredients, except the salad leaves, to the slow cooker. Combine well, cover and leave to cook on high for 3-4 hours or until the chicken is cooked through and the carrots are tender.
- Cut the chicken breasts into thick diagonal slices and pour the olives, juices and vegetables over the top.
- Serve with the salad leaves for a delicious warm salad.

You could also serve this with rice or noodles if you are feeling particularly hungry.

Ingredients:

4 x skinless chicken breasts each weighing 125g/4oz
1 tsp turmeric
½ tsp ground cinnamon
2 onions, sliced
2 lemons, sliced
2 carrots, cut into thin batons
1 garlic clove, crushed
1 tbsp runny honey
½ tbsp freshly grated ginger
75g/3oz pitted kalamata olives
370ml/1½ cups chicken stock/broth
4 tbsp freshly chopped coriander/cilantro
200g/7oz mixed salad leaves
Salt & pepper to taste

Harissa Chicken
Serves 4

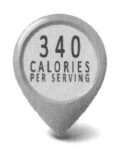

340 CALORIES PER SERVING

Ingredients:

**4 x skinless chicken breasts
each weighing 125g/4oz
1 tsp each turmeric &
cumin
½ tsp ground cinnamon
75g/3oz dried apricots,
chopped
1 tsp harissa paste
1 tbsp lemon juice
2 tbsp tomato puree
1 onion, sliced
2 red (bell) peppers, thinly
sliced
2 garlic cloves, crushed
1 tbsp runny honey
250ml/1 cup chicken
stock/broth
200g/7oz long grain rice
1 lemon, cut into wedges
Salt & pepper to taste**

Method:

• Season the chicken breasts.
• Add all the ingredients, except the rice & lemon wedges, to the slow cooker. Combine well, cover and leave to cook on high for 3-4 hours or until the chicken is cooked through.
• Meanwhile cook the rice in salted boiling water until tender.
• Cut the chicken breasts into thick diagonal slices and serve with the drained rice and lemon wedges.

Harissa is a Tunisian hot chilli sauce readily available in most supermarkets.

44

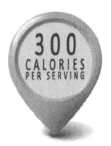

300 CALORIES PER SERVING

Roasted Garlic Chicken
Serves 4

Method:

- Season the chicken breasts.
- Separate the garlic cloves but don't peel them.
- Add all the ingredients, except the spring onions, broad beans & spinach, to the slow cooker. Cover and leave to cook on low for 3-4 hours.
- Add the rest of the ingredients to the slow cooker, increase the heat to high and cook for a further 2-3 hours or until the chicken is cooked through and the vegetables are tender.
- Serve with the whole garlic cloves arranged on the plates.

Ingredients:

4 x skinless chicken breasts each weighing 125g/4oz
2 whole heads of garlic
1 onion, sliced
120ml/½ cup chicken stock/broth
1 lemon, cut into wedges
1 large bunch spring onions/scallions, green tops trimmed
400g/14oz tinned broad beans
150g/5oz spinach
Salt & pepper to taste

The garlic in this dish is not nearly as overpowering as you might imagine.

Thai Chicken
Serves 4

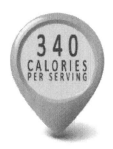

340 CALORIES PER SERVING

Ingredients:

**4 x skinless chicken breasts
each weighing 125g/4oz
4 garlic cloves, crushed
1 onion, sliced
2 lemongrass stalks, finely
chopped
1 tsp ground coriander/
cilantro
2 tbsp Thai fish sauce
1 tbsp coconut cream
2 tbsp soy sauce
120ml/½ cup chicken
stock/broth
200g/7oz fine egg noodles
4 tbsp freshly chopped
coriander/cilantro
1 small bunch spring
onions/scallions, sliced
Salt & pepper to taste**

Method:

• Season the chicken breasts.
• Add all the ingredients, except the noodles, fresh coriander & spring onions, to the slow cooker. Cover and leave to cook on high for 3-4 hours or until the chicken is cooked through.
• Meanwhile cook the egg noodles in salted boiling water until tender.
• Cut the chicken breasts thinly and serve with the drained noodles, sprinkled with spring onions and chopped coriander.

You could also add some crushed chilli flakes to this dish if you like.

46

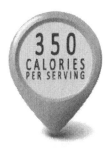

350 CALORIES PER SERVING

Spicy Chicken & Peppers
Serves 4

Method:

- Season the chicken.
- Mix the cornflour with a little warm water to make a paste.
- Add this to the chopped tomatoes and chicken stock.
- Add all the ingredients, except the rice & fresh coriander to the slow cooker. Cover and leave to cook on high for 3-5 hours or until the chicken is cooked through.
- Meanwhile cook the rice in salted boiling water until tender.
- Serve the spicy chicken on top of the drained rice sprinkled with chopped coriander.

The cornflour paste should ensure this dish has a nice thick sauce. Add a little more if needed.

Ingredients:

**500g/1lb 2oz skinless chicken breasts, cubed
2 tsp cornflour
2 red (bell) peppers, sliced
1 green (bell) pepper, sliced
2 garlic cloves, crushed
2 onions, sliced
1 tbsp freshly grated ginger
1 tsp each ground coriander/cilantro, turmeric & chilli powder
½ tsp each salt & brown sugar
400g/14oz tinned chopped tomatoes
60ml/¼ cup chicken stock/broth
200g/7oz fine basmati rice
4 tbsp freshly chopped coriander/cilantro
Salt & pepper to taste**

Hot Chicken Skewers
Serves 4

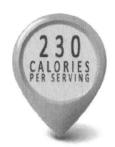

230 CALORIES PER SERVING

Ingredients:

500g/1lb 2oz skinless chicken breasts, cubed
1 tsp crushed chilli flakes
2 garlic cloves, crushed
2 tbsp soy sauce
2 tbsp lemon juice
½ tsp each salt & brown sugar
2 onions, sliced
60ml/¼ cup chicken stock/ broth
2 romaine lettuces, shredded
4 tbsp fat free Greek yoghurt
Wooden kebab skewers
Low cal cooking oil spray
Salt & pepper to taste

Method:

• Season the chicken.
• Mix together the chilli flakes, garlic, soy sauce, lemon juice, salt & sugar to make a marinade.
• Place the chicken and marinade in a bowl and mix well. Ideally you would leave to marinade for a few hours or overnight but don't worry if you don't have time.
• Gently sauté the onions in a little low cal spray until soft.
• Skewer the chicken pieces on the wooden sticks and place in the slow cooker along with the sautéd onions and stock. Cover and leave to cook on high for 2-3 hours or until the chicken is cooked through.
• Serve the skewers with shredded lettuce and a dollop of yoghurt on the side.

You could also add button mushrooms and cherry tomatoes to cook on the skewers if you want to mix things up a little.

48

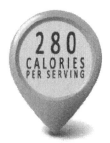

280 CALORIES PER SERVING

Teryaki Chicken
Serves 4

Method:

- Season the chicken.
- Mix together the soy sauce, brown sugar, garlic & sesame oil to make a marinade.
- Place the chicken and marinade in a bowl and mix well.
- Skewer the chicken pieces on the wooden sticks and place in the slow cooker along with the stock. Cover and leave to cook on high for 2-3 hours or until the chicken is cooked through.
- Meanwhile cook the rice in salted boiling water until tender.
- Serve the skewers and drained rice sprinkled with chopped spring onions.

Ingredients:

500g/1lb 2oz skinless chicken breasts, cubed
60ml/¼ cup soy sauce
2 tsp brown sugar
3 garlic cloves, crushed
2 tbsp sesame oil
60ml/¼ cup chicken stock/ broth
Wooden kebab skewers
200g/7oz basmati rice
Large bunch spring onions/ scallions, chopped
Salt & pepper to taste

This is a lovely sweet dish. You could add some lemon wedges when you serve if you wish.

Chicken & Pineapple
Serves 4

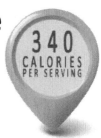

340 CALORIES PER SERVING

Ingredients:

**500g/1lb 2oz skinless
chicken breasts, cubed
2 tsp cornflour
1 red (bell) pepper, sliced
2 carrots, cut into
matchsticks
2 garlic cloves, crushed
1 onion, sliced
3 tbsp soy sauce
200g/7oz tinned pineapple
60ml/¼ cup pineapple
juice
120ml/½ cup chicken
stock/broth
200g/7oz fine egg noodles
1 bunch spring onions,
sliced lengthways
Salt & pepper to taste**

Method:

• Season the chicken.
• Mix the cornflour with a little warm water to make a paste. Add this to the chicken stock and pineapple juice.
• Add all the ingredients, except the egg noodles & spring onions, to the slow cooker. Cover and leave to cook on high for 3-4 hours or until the chicken is cooked through.
• Meanwhile cook the noodles in salted boiling water until tender.
• Serve the chicken and drained egg noodles with the sliced spring onions.

You could add the pineapple much later in the cooking if you prefer.

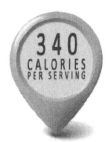

340 CALORIES PER SERVING

Coronation Chicken
Serves 4

Method:

- Season the chicken.
- Gently sauté the onion, carrots & garlic in a little low cal oil for a few minutes until softened.
- Add all the ingredients, except the watercress, yoghurt & rice, to the slow cooker. Cover and leave to cook on high for 3-4 hours or until the chicken is cooked through.
- Meanwhile cook the rice in salted boiling water until tender.
- Stir the yoghurt and watercress through the chicken until the yoghurt is warmed through and the watercress is wilted.
- Serve with the drained rice.

Ingredients:

500g/1lb 2oz skinless chicken breasts, cubed
1 onion, sliced
2 carrots, cut into matchsticks
2 garlic cloves, crushed
1 tbsp curry powder
1 tbsp tomato puree/paste
75g/3oz sultanas
120ml/½ cup chicken stock/broth
200g/7oz watercress
3 tbsp fat free Greek yoghurt
200g/7oz basmati rice
Low cal cooking oil spray
Salt & pepper to taste

Mild curry powder works well with the recipe but you could go hotter if you prefer.

51

Italian Chicken
Serves 4

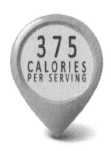

375 CALORIES PER SERVING

Ingredients:

500g/1lb 2oz skinless chicken breasts, cubed
2 red (bell) peppers, sliced
1 onion, sliced
2 carrots, cut into matchsticks
2 garlic cloves, crushed
400g/14oz tinned cannellini beans, drained
120ml/½ cup tomato passata/sieved tomatoes
200g/7oz tenderstem broccoli
60ml/¼ cup chicken stock/broth
4 tbsp freshly chopped flat leaf parsley
1 lemon, cut into wedges
Low cal cooking oil spray
Salt & pepper to taste

Method:

• Season the chicken.
• Gently sauté the peppers, onion, carrots & garlic in a little low cal oil for a few minutes until softened.
• Add all the ingredients, except the parsley & lemon, to the slow cooker. Cover and leave to cook on high for 3-5 hours or until the chicken is cooked through.
• Sprinkle with chopped parsley and serve with lemon wedges.

You could use spinach or kale rather than broccoli if you prefer.

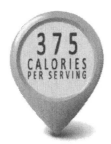

375 CALORIES PER SERVING

Chicken & Prawn Stew
Serves 4

Method:

- Season the chicken and prawns.
- Gently sauté the peppers, onion & garlic in a little low cal oil for a few minutes until softened.
- Add all the ingredients to the slow cooker. Cover and leave to cook on high for 3-5 hours or until the chicken and prawns are cooked through.
- Meanwhile cook the rice in salted boiling water until tender.
- Drain and serve with the chicken stew.

Ingredients:

250g/9oz skinless chicken breasts, cubed
250g/9oz raw king prawns
2 red (bell) peppers, sliced
1 onion, sliced
2 garlic cloves, crushed
60ml/¼ cup low fat coconut milk
60ml/¼ cup chicken stock/broth
50g/2oz cashew nuts, chopped
½ tsp salt
3 tbsp lime juice
200g/7oz long grain rice
Low cal cooking oil spray
Salt & pepper to taste

Lime wedges and chopped parsley are good additional garnishes for this dish too.

Tarragon Chicken
Serves 4

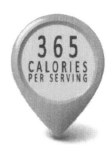

365 CALORIES PER SERVING

Ingredients:

4 x skinless chicken breasts each weighing 125g/4oz
50g/2oz lean, back bacon, chopped
2 leeks, chopped
1 onion, sliced
2 garlic cloves, crushed
2 carrots, sliced
1 tsp English mustard
120ml/½ cup dry cider
120ml/½ cup chicken stock/broth
3 tbsp freshly chopped tarragon
400g/14oz asparagus spears
2 tbsp low fat crème fraiche
Low cal cooking oil spray
Salt & pepper to taste

Method:

• Season the chicken.
• Gently sauté the bacon, leeks, onion & garlic in a little low cal oil for a few minutes until softened.
• Add all the ingredients, except the crème fraiche, to the slow cooker. Cover and leave to cook on high for 3-5 hours or until the chicken is cooked through.
• Remove the chicken breasts, stir through the crème fraiche and pour the creamy sauce over the chicken breasts to serve.

If you prefer a thicker sauce you could add a little cornflour dissolved in warm water during cooking.

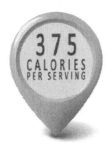

375 CALORIES PER SERVING

Pomegranate Chicken
Serves 4

Method:

- Season the chicken.
- Cut the pomegranates in half and bang each one hard on the back to release all the seeds.
- Place all the pomegranate seeds in a bowl with the sugar and mix well.
- Gently sauté the onion and garlic in a little low cal oil for a few minutes until softened.
- Add all the ingredients, except the beansprouts, parsley & lemon, to the slow cooker. Cover and leave to cook on high for 3-5 hours or until the chicken is cooked through.
- Half an hour before the end of cooking time add the beansprouts and stir.
- When the beansprouts are tender sprinkle with chopped parsley and serve with the lemon wedges.

Add a little more brown sugar if you feel the dish needs additional sweetness.

Ingredients:

500g/1lb 2oz skinless chicken breasts, cubed
2 pomegranates
2 tsp brown sugar
1 onion, sliced
2 garlic cloves, crushed
½ tsp each turmeric & ground cinnamon
250ml/1 cup chicken stock/broth
200g/7oz green beans
100g/7oz beansprouts
4 tbsp freshly chopped flat leaf parsley
1 lemon, cut into wedges
Salt & pepper to taste

Peanut Butter Chicken
Serves 4

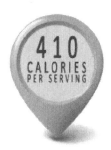

410 CALORIES PER SERVING

Ingredients:

500g/1lb 2oz skinless
chicken breasts, cubed
3 tbsp smooth peanut
butter
1 onion, sliced
2 garlic cloves, crushed
1 tbsp freshly grated
ginger
2 tsp paprika
250ml/1 cup tomato
pasatta/sieved tomatoes
2 tbsp worcestershire
sauce
150g/5oz vine ripened
tomatoes, chopped
4 tbsp freshly chopped flat
leaf parsley
200g/7oz gnocchi
Salt & pepper to taste

Method:

• Season the chicken and mix with the peanut butter.
• Add all the ingredients, except the gnocchi & parsley, to the slow cooker. Cover and leave to cook on high for 3-5 hours or until the chicken is cooked through.
• Meanwhile cook the gnocchi in salted boiling water until tender.
• Serve the chicken and gnocchi with the parsley sprinkled over the top.

You could add the gnocchi to the slow cooker to cook for 20-30 minutes if you prefer to have everything ready in the same pot.

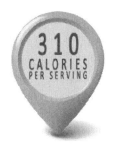

310 CALORIES PER SERVING

Sauerkraut Chicken Stew
Serves 4

Method:

• Season the chicken.

• Gently sauté the mushrooms, onion, garlic & sausages in a little low cal oil for a few minutes.

• Slice the sausages into thick 1 inch/2cm pieces.

• Add all the ingredients to the slow cooker. Cover and leave to cook on high for 3-5 hours or until the chicken and sausages are cooked through.

Ingredients:

400g/14oz skinless chicken breasts, cubed
200g/7oz mushrooms, sliced
1 onion, sliced
2 garlic cloves, crushed
250g/9oz lean sausages
2 apples, cored and sliced
370ml/1½ cups chicken stock/broth
250g/9oz sauerkraut
200g/7oz green cabbage, shredded
Salt & pepper to taste

This is a soupy stew which is lovely served in bowls with crusty bread to mop up the juices.

Fish

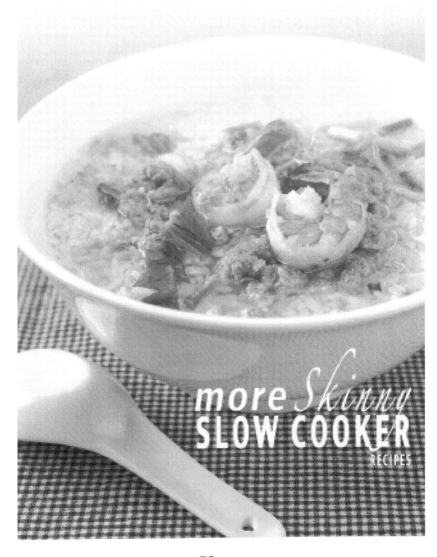

Baby Courgettes, Tuna & Rocket
Serves 4

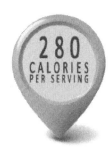

Ingredients:

500g/1lb 2oz skinless, boneless fresh tuna fillets, cubed
300g/11oz baby courgettes/zucchini
2 garlic cloves, crushed
1 onion, sliced
200g/7oz vine ripened tomatoes, chopped
4 tbsp freshly chopped flat leaf parsley
2 tbsp sundried tomato puree/paste
60ml/¼ cup fish or vegetable stock/broth
125g/4oz rocket leaves
Low cal cooking oil spray
Salt & pepper to taste

Method:

• Season the fish fillets.
• Cut the courgettes in half lengthways.
• Gently sauté the garlic, onions, chopped tomatoes and courgettes in a little low cal spray for a few minutes until softened.
• Place all the ingredients, except the rocket, in the slow cooker. Combine gently, season, cover and leave to cook on high for 1-2 hours or until the tuna is cooked through.
• At the end of the cooking time add the rocket and gently fold through the dish just once.
• Serve immediately in shallow bowls.

Adding the rocket right at the end of cooking will wilt it slightly as it warms through. If you prefer your rocket crunchy, serve on the side instead.

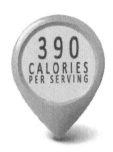

390
CALORIES
PER SERVING

Creamy Haddock & New Potatoes
Serves 4

Method:

- Season the haddock fillets.
- Gently sauté the onions, leeks, carrots & garlic in a little low cal spray for a few minutes.
- Add all the ingredients, except the cream, parsley & lemon, to the slow cooker. Combine well, cover and leave to cook on high for 2-3 hours or until the fish is cooked through and the potatoes are tender.
- Stir through the cream and leave to warm for a minute or two.
- Serve in bowls sprinkled with fresh parsley and lemon wedges on the side.

Ingredients:

500g/1lb 2oz skinless, boneless smoked haddock fillets, cubed
1 onion, chopped
1 leek, sliced
2 carrots, sliced
1 garlic clove, crushed
400g/14oz new potatoes, quartered
120ml/½ cup fish or vegetable stock/broth
200g/7oz spinach, chopped
60ml/¼ cup single cream
2 tbsp freshly chopped flat leaf parsley
1 lemon, cut into wedges
Low cal cooking oil spray
Salt & pepper to taste

Using traditional yellow-dyed smoked haddock gives this dish a great colour but you can use any smoked fish you prefer.

61

Monkfish & Tomato Stew
Serves 4

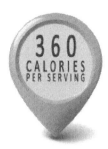

360 CALORIES PER SERVING

Ingredients:

500g/1lb 2oz skinless, boneless monkfish fillets, cubed
1 onion, chopped
1 tsp djion mustard
400g/14oz tinned chopped tomatoes
2 garlic cloves, crushed
2 tbsp tomato puree/paste
1 tsp crushed black pepper
1 tsp dried oregano
1 bayleaf
½ tsp each salt & brown sugar
4 tbsp freshly chopped flat leaf parsley
200g/7oz long grain rice
Salt & pepper to taste

Method:

• Season the monkfish fillets.
• Add all the ingredients, except the rice, to the slow cooker. Combine gently, season, cover and leave to cook on high for 1-2 hours or until the fish is cooked through.
• Meanwhile cook the rice in salted boiling water until tender.
• Divide the drained rice into bowls and serve the fish stew over the top of the rice.

It's possible to cook the rice in the slow cooker if you prefer. Add the rice and 250ml/1 cup of extra stock to the slow cooker about 20-30 minutes before the cooking time is over.

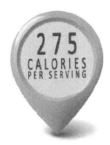

275
CALORIES
PER SERVING

Coconut Cod Stew
Serves 4

Method:

- Season the cod fillets.
- Add all the ingredients, except the lime wedges, to the slow cooker. Combine gently, cover and leave to cook on high for 1-2 hours or until the fish is cooked through.
- Spoon into shallow bowls and serve with lime wedges on the side.

Ingredients:

500g/1lb 2oz skinless, boneless cod fillets, cubed
2 onions, chopped
1 green chilli, deseeded and finely chopped
400g/14oz tinned chopped tomatoes
2 garlic cloves, crushed
½ tsp ground allspice
2 tbsp tomato puree/paste
½ tsp each salt & brown sugar
120ml/½ cup low fat coconut milk
4 tbsp freshly chopped flat leaf parsley
200g/7oz mushrooms, sliced
200g/7oz French beans
1 lime, cut into wedges
Salt & pepper to taste

A whole green chilli may be too spicy for some palates so adjust to suit your own taste.

Chinese Spiced Fish
Serves 4

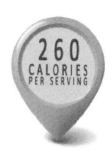

260 CALORIES PER SERVING

Ingredients:

500g/1lb 2oz skinless, boneless cod or haddock fillets, cubed
2 tsp Chinese five-spice powder
1 tbsp plain/all purpose flour
2 onions, chopped
1 tsp each ground ginger & brown sugar
250ml/1 cup fish or vegetable stock/broth
2 garlic cloves, crushed
150g/5oz baby sweetcorn, sliced
150g/5oz mangetout, roughly chopped
2 tbsp soy sauce
200g/7oz beansprouts
Salt & pepper to taste

Method:

• Season the fish fillets.
• Place the fish pieces in a small plastic bag with the flour and Chinese five-spice. Shake well to cover each fish piece in flour & spice.
• Place the floured fish in the slow cooker along with all the other ingredients, except the beansprouts.
• Combine gently, season, cover and leave to cook on high for 1-2 hours or until the fish is cooked through.
• 5 minutes before the end of cooking time add the beansprouts.
• Combine and serve immediately.

Add more five-spice to this dish if you are keen on its unique oriental taste.

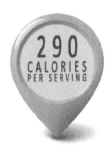

290
CALORIES
PER SERVING

Monkfish & Olive Stew
Serves 4

Method:

- Season the fish fillets.
- Place the fish pieces in a small plastic bag with the flour, turmeric & coriander. Shake well to cover each fish piece in flour & spice.
- Meanwhile gently sauté the onions and garlic in a little low cal spray for a few minutes until softened.
- Place the floured fish in the slow cooker along with all the other ingredients, except the rocket leaves. Combine gently, cover and leave to cook on high for 1-2 hours or until the fish is cooked through.
- Serve in shallow bowls on a bed of rocket.

Ingredients:

500g/1lb 2oz skinless, boneless monkfish fillets
½ tsp each turmeric & coriander/cilantro
1 tbsp plain/all purpose flour
2 onions, sliced
2 garlic cloves, crushed
60ml/¼ cup fish or vegetable stock/broth
150g/5oz vine ripened tomatoes, chopped
2 handfuls black pitted olives
200g/7oz rocket
Low cal cooking oil spray
Salt & pepper to taste

Monkfish can be expensive so feel free to use any other meaty white fish you prefer.

Lemon Sole With Orange Slices
Serves 4

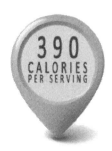

390 CALORIES PER SERVING

Ingredients:

500g/1lb 2oz skinless, boneless lemon sole fillets
1 orange
50g/2oz drained anchovy fillets
2 garlic cloves, crushed
1 onion, sliced
½ tsp ground black pepper
60ml/¼ cup vegetable stock/broth
1 large bunch freshly chopped basil
2 romaine lettuces, shredded
2 ripe avocados, de-stoned and sliced
Low cal cooking oil spray
Salt & pepper to taste

Method:

• Season the fish fillets.
• Peel the orange of its skin and pith. Slice as thinly as possible.
• Gently sauté the anchovies, garlic & onions in a little low cal spray for a few minutes until softened.
• Place all the ingredients, except the shredded lettuce & avocados in the slow cooker. Combine gently, season, cover and leave to cook on high for 1-2 hours or until the sole is cooked through.
• Serve on plates with the shredded lettuce and sliced avocados on the side.

The anchovies in this recipe give the dish a lovely salty depth.

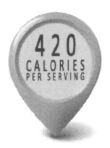

420 CALORIES PER SERVING

Fish Gratin
Serves 4

Method:

• Season the fish fillets.
• Gently sauté the garlic, onions and potato slices in a little low cal spray for a few minutes until softened.
• Place all the ingredients in the slow cooker adding the fish first, finishing with the potatoes layered on top and the cheese sprinkled over.
• Season, cover and leave to cook on high for 2-4 hours or until the fish is cooked through and the potatoes are tender.

Ingredients:

500g/1lb 2oz skinless, boneless haddock fillets, cubed
2 garlic cloves, crushed
2 onions, sliced
400g/14oz potatoes, thinly sliced
200g/7oz spinach, chopped
½ tsp ground black pepper
60ml/¼ cup fish or vegetable stock/broth
4 tbsp freshly chopped basil
50g/2oz low fat grated cheddar cheese
Low cal cooking oil spray
Salt & pepper to taste

You could replace the basil in this recipe with fresh thyme as an alternative taste.

Fresh Herb Fish Stew
Serves 4

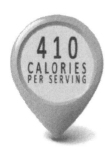

410 CALORIES PER SERVING

Ingredients:

500g/1lb 2oz skinless, boneless white fish fillets, cubed
2 garlic cloves, crushed
1 red onion, sliced
400g/7oz potatoes, cubed
200g/7oz vine ripened tomatoes, chopped
200g/7oz spinach, chopped
60ml/¼ cup fish or vegetable stock/broth
3 bunches of chopped fresh herbs
1 tsp paprika
2 tbsp lime juice
Low cal cooking oil spray
Salt & pepper to taste

Method:

• Season the fish fillets.
• Gently sauté the garlic, red onions, potatoes & chopped tomatoes in a little low cal spray for a few minutes until softened.
• Place all the ingredients in the slow cooker. Combine gently, season, cover and leave to cook on high for 2-4 hours or until the fish is cooked through and the potatoes are tender.

You can experiment with fresh herb combinations but a bunch each of freshly chopped flat leaf parsley, basil & coriander/ cilantro is a great place to start.

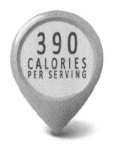

390
CALORIES
PER SERVING

Spicy Ginger Fish
Serves 4

Method:

- Season the fish fillets.
- Mix together the coriander, grated ginger, tomato puree, salt & sweet chilli sauce to make a paste. Place in a bowl with the fish fillets and cover the fish in the paste.
- Gently sauté the garlic, onions & chopped tomatoes in a little low cal spray for a few minutes until softened.
- Place all the ingredients, except the noodles and lime wedges, in the slow cooker. Combine gently, cover and leave to cook on high for 1-2 hours or until the fish is cooked through.
- Meanwhile cook the noodles in salted boiling water until tender. Drain and serve in shallow bowls with the fish & sauce spooned on top and lime wedges on the side.

You could also add a small chopped red chilli to this dish if you prefer more spice.

Ingredients:

500g/1lb 2oz skinless, boneless white fish fillets, cubed
2 tbsp freshly chopped coriander/cilantro
1 tbsp freshly grated ginger
2 tbsp tomato puree/paste
1 tsp salt
1 tbsp sweet chilli sauce
2 garlic cloves, crushed
1 onion, sliced
200g/7oz vine ripened tomatoes, chopped
60ml/¼ cup fish or vegetable stock/broth
200g/7oz fine egg noodles
1 lime, cut into wedges
Low cal cooking oil spray
Salt & pepper to taste

Lemongrass Fish & Noodles
Serves 4

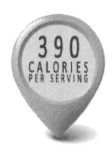

Ingredients:

500g/1lb 2oz skinless, boneless fresh white fish fillets, cubed
2 lemongrass stalks, finely chopped
2 garlic cloves, crushed
2 onions, chopped
1 red chilli, deseeded and finely chopped
1 tsp turmeric
120ml/½ cup coconut cream
125g/4oz peas
200g/7oz tinned chopped tomatoes
200g/7oz ready-to-eat bamboo shoots
2 free range eggs
200g/7oz fine egg noodles
Low cal cooking oil spray
Salt & pepper to taste

Method:

• Season the fish fillets.
• Gently sauté the chopped lemongrass, garlic, onions, chilli and turmeric in a little low cal spray for a few minutes until softened.
• Place all the ingredients, except the eggs and noodles, in the slow cooker. Combine gently, season, cover and leave to cook on high for 1-2 hours or until the fish is cooked through.
• Meanwhile hard-boil the eggs. Peel and cut into quarters.
• Cook the noodles in salted boiling water until tender.
• Serve the fish & sauce spooned on top of the noodles in shallow bowls with two boiled egg quarters on the top of each bowl.

This dish is also lovely with chopped spring onions and lime wedges as a garnish.

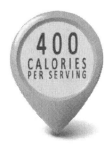

400 CALORIES PER SERVING

Trout & Creamy Mushrooms
Serves 4

Method:

- Season the fish fillets.
- Gently sauté the mushrooms, garlic and onions in a little low cal spray for a few minutes until softened. Remove from the heat and stir through the crème fraiche.
- Place all the ingredients, except the rice, parsley and lemon, in the slow cooker. Combine gently, cover and leave to cook on high for 1-2 hours or until the fish is cooked through.
- Meanwhile cook the rice in salted boiling water until tender.
- Serve the whole fillets and mushrooms on plates with the rice on the side.
- Sprinkle the parsley over the rice and add a wedge of lemon to serve.

Ingredients:

500g/1lb 2oz skinless, boneless trout fillets
450g/1lb mushrooms, sliced
2 garlic cloves, crushed
1 onion, chopped
250ml/1 cup low fat crème fraiche
150g/5oz petit pois peas
½ tsp freshly ground black pepper
60ml/¼ cup fish or vegetable stock/broth
200g/7oz long grain rice
2 tbsp freshly chopped flat leaf parsley
1 lemon, cut into wedges
Low cal cooking oil spray
Salt & pepper to taste

Add a little water to the sauté pan if you find the low cal spray isn't oily enough to move the mushrooms around the pan.

Coriander & Mint Curry
Serves 4

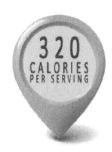

320 CALORIES PER SERVING

Ingredients:

500g/1lb 2oz skinless, boneless white fish fillets
1 tsp each coriander/ cilantro seeds & cumin seeds
2 garlic cloves, crushed
1 onion, sliced
1 bunch spring onions/ scallions, chopped
1 tsp each ground turmeric & paprika
3 tbsp freshly chopped coriander/cilantro
3 tbsp freshly chopped mint
3 tbsp freshly chopped flat leaf parsley
150g/5oz peas
120ml/½ cup low fat coconut milk
120ml/½ cup tomato passata/sieved tomatoes
200g/7oz basmati rice

Method:

• Season the fish fillets.
• Grind the cumin and coriander seeds in a pestle & mortar.
• Gently sauté the garlic, onions, spring onions & crushed seeds in a little low cal spray for a few minutes until softened.
• Place all the ingredients, except the rice, in the slow cooker. Combine gently, cover and leave to cook on high for 1-2 hours or until the fish is cooked through.
• Meanwhile cook the rice in salted boiling water until tender.
• Drain and serve the fish on a bed of rice.

The chopped herbs in this dish give it a lovely fresh taste. Reserve a little for garnish when you serve.

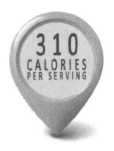

310
CALORIES
PER SERVING

Pineapple & Fish Stew
Serves 4

Method:

- Season the fish fillets.
- Mix the cornflour with a little warm water to form a paste.
- Place all the ingredients, except the noodles & parsley, in the slow cooker.
- Combine gently, cover and leave to cook on high for 1-2 hours or until the fish is cooked through.
- Meanwhile cook the noodles in salted boiling water until tender.
- Serve sprinkled with parsley on a bed of noodles.

Ingredients:

500g/1lb 2oz skinless, boneless white fish fillets
2 tsp cornflour
2 carrots, cut into batons
1 yellow (bell) pepper, sliced
200g/7oz baby sweetcorn, sliced
1 onion, sliced
2 garlic cloves, crushed
½ peeled pineapple, flesh cubed
250ml/1 cup fish or vegetable stock/broth
150g/5oz peas
200g/7oz fine egg noodles
3 tbsp freshly chopped flat leaf parsley
Low cal cooking oil spray
Salt & pepper to taste

You could hold off adding the pineapple chunks until 10 minutes before the end of cooking time if you prefer it crunchy.

Garam Masala Prawns
Serves 4

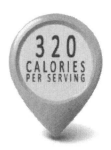

320 CALORIES PER SERVING

Ingredients:

700g/1lb 9oz raw king prawns
2 tsp garam masala
½ tsp salt
150g/5oz potatoes, cubed
250g/9oz peas
1 onion, sliced
2 garlic cloves, crushed
1 tsp each turmeric, cumin, coriander/cilantro & paprika
½ tsp cayenne peppers
400g/14oz tinned chopped tomatoes
2 tbsp fat free Greek yoghurt
200g/7oz basmati rice
3 tbsp freshly chopped coriander
Low cal cooking oil spray
Salt & pepper to taste

Method:

• Coat the prawns in garam masala & salt.
• Place all the ingredients, except the yoghurt, rice & chopped coriander, in the slow cooker.
• Combine gently, cover and leave to cook on high for 2-3 hours or until the prawns are cooked through and the potatoes are tender.
• Meanwhile cook the rice in salted boiling water until tender.
• Add the yoghurt to the slow cooker and stir to gently warm through.
• Serve with the drained rice and chopped coriander.

Fenugreek seeds and mint are also good alternatives to add to this dish instead of coriander.

Vegetable

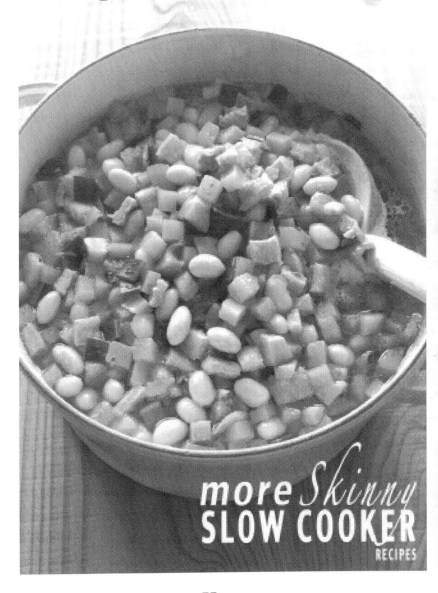

more *Skinny*
SLOW COOKER
RECIPES

Celery & Lentil Casserole
Serves 4

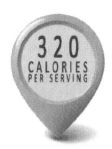

320 CALORIES PER SERVING

Ingredients:

2 leeks, sliced
1 onion, sliced
2 garlic cloves, crushed
2 tsp cornflour
370ml/1½ cups vegetable stock/broth
2 carrots, cut into batons
6 stalks celery, quartered
2 parsnips, chopped
200g/7oz sweet potatoes, cubed
200g/7oz lentils
1 tsp dried thyme
1 bunch freshly chopped basil
Low cal cooking oil spray
Salt & pepper to taste

Method:

• Gently sauté the leeks, onion and garlic in a little low cal spray for a few minutes until softened.
• Mix the cornflour with a little warm water to make a paste. Add this paste to the stock and stir well.
• Place all the ingredients in the slow cooker. Combine gently, cover and leave to cook on high for 2-4 hours or until the vegetables and lentils are tender.
• Season and serve in shallow bowls.

Add more stock if the dish is too dry. Conversely if you need to thicken it up, take the lid off and continue to cook for a little longer while the sauce reduces down.

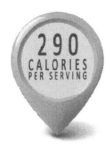

290
CALORIES
PER SERVING

Mozzarella & Baby Vegetable Bake

Serves 4

Method:

• Cut all the baby vegetables, mushrooms, tomatoes and olives in half lengthways and gently sauté them with the garlic and olive oil for 5-10 minutes until softened.
• Stir through the dried mixed herbs & balsamic vinegar and remove from the heat.
• Place all the ingredients, except the parsley, in the slow cooker. Combine gently, season, cover and leave to cook on high for 2-4 hours or until the vegetables are tender.
• Sprinkle with chopped parsley and serve in shallow bowls.

Ingredients:

1.25kg/2¾lb mix of baby courgettes/zucchini, aubergine/eggplant, sweetcorn, shallots, button mushrooms & cherry tomatoes
1 handful pitted black olives
2 garlic cloves, crushed
1 tbsp olive oil
2 tsp dried mixed herbs
2 tbsp balsamic vinegar
60ml/¼ cup vegetable stock
150g/5oz low fat grated mozzarella cheese
4 tbsp freshly chopped flat leaf parsley
Salt & pepper to taste

This should be a fairly dry 'roasted' dish. However you don't want it to dry up too much so add a little more water or stock during cooking if needed.

Spinach Borlotti Beans
Serves 4

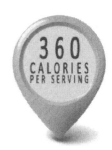

360 CALORIES PER SERVING

Ingredients:

800g/1 ¾lb tinned borlotti beans, drained
400g/14oz spinach
200g/7oz vine-ripened tomatoes, quartered
60ml/¼ cup vegetable stock/broth
1 small handful pine nuts
1 small handful raisins
1 garlic clove, crushed
1 tsp each cumin & paprika
½ tsp each brown sugar & salt
1 lemon, cut into wedges
1 bunch freshly chopped flat leaf parsley
Salt & pepper to taste

Method:

• Place all the ingredients, except the lemon & parsley, in the slow cooker. Combine gently, season, cover and leave to cook on high for 1-2 hours or until the vegetables are tender.
• Sprinkle with chopped parsley and serve in shallow bowls with lemon wedges.

You could also use flageolet, chickpeas or haricot beans for this recipe if you prefer.

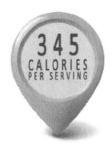

345 CALORIES PER SERVING

Roasted Vegetable Penne
Serves 4

Method:

• Place all the ingredients, except the penne, balsamic vinegar & olive oil, in the slow cooker. Combine gently, season, cover and leave to cook on high for 2-3 hours or until the vegetables are tender (add a little more stock during cooking if needed).
• Meanwhile cook the penne in salted boiling water until tender.
• Toss the cooked vegetables & penne together along with the olive oil and balsamic vinegar.
• Season well and serve.

Ingredients:

2 red (bell) peppers, quartered
1 aubergine/eggplant, sliced
2 red onions, cut into wedges
150g/5oz courgettes/zucchini, sliced
150g/5oz portabella mushrooms, sliced
250g/9oz asparagus tips, roughly chopped
60ml/¼ cup vegetable stock/broth
2 garlic cloves, crushed
1 bunch freshly chopped basil leaves
200g/7oz penne pasta
3 tbsp balsamic vinegar
2 tbsp olive oil
Salt & pepper to taste

Fusilli and farfalle pasta will work just as well in this recipe.

Vegetables & Cashew Nuts
Serves 4

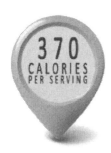

Ingredients:

1 onion, sliced
1 tbsp freshly grated ginger
2 garlic cloves, crushed
4 carrots, cut into thin matchsticks
1 red (bell) pepper, sliced
1 bunch spring onions/ scallions, sliced lengthways
150g/5oz baby sweetcorn
125g/4oz plain cashew nuts
150g/5oz chestnut mushrooms, sliced
60ml/¼ cup vegetable stock/broth
3 tbsp soy sauce
200g/7oz fine egg noodles
1 cucumber, finely chopped
1 tbsp sesame oil
Low cal cooking oil spray
Salt & pepper to taste

Method:

• Gently sauté the onions, ginger and garlic in a little low cal oil for a few minutes until softened.
• Place all the ingredients, except the noodles, cucumber and sesame oil, in the slow cooker. Combine gently, season, cover and leave to cook on high for 1-2 hours or until the vegetables are tender.
• Meanwhile cook the egg noodles in salted boiling water until tender.
• Toss the cooked vegetables, drained noodles and sesame oil together.
• Add the cucumber, quickly toss through and serve immediately.

Adding the cucumber to this dish gives the meal a lovely fresh 'bite'.

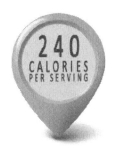

240
CALORIES
PER SERVING

Shredded Red Cabbage In Pomegranate Juice

Serves 4

Method:

• Place all the ingredients in the slow cooker. Combine gently, cover and leave to cook on high for 3-4 hours or until the vegetables are tender.
• Season well with salt and lots of black pepper before serving.

Ingredients:

2 red cabbages, shredded
2 red onions, sliced
1 fennel bulb, chopped
2 Granny Smith apples, cored and sliced
75g/3oz raisins
250ml/1 cup pomegranate juice
Salt & pepper to taste

You could use apple juice rather than pomegranate juice in this recipe if you like.

Leeks, Lentils & Baked Eggs
Serves 4

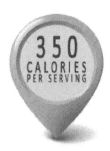

350 CALORIES PER SERVING

Ingredients:

300g/9oz lentils
1 onion, sliced
3 leeks, sliced
1 tsp each ground coriander/cilantro & turmeric
750ml/3 cups vegetable stock/broth
4 free range eggs
4 tbsp freshly chopped flat leaf parsley
Salt & pepper to taste

Method:

• Place all the ingredients, except the eggs and parsley, in the slow cooker.
• Combine gently, season, cover and leave to cook on high for 3-5 hours or until the lentils are soft and the stock has been absorbed (add more stock if needed).
• Half an hour before the end of cooking make 4 'wells' in the lentils and crack an egg into each well.
• When the eggs are firm, serve and sprinkle with chopped parsley.

Use whichever combination of lentils you prefer for this dish. Chopped coriander makes a good additional garnish too.

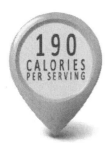

190 CALORIES PER SERVING

Cauliflower & Broccoli Bake
Serves 4

Method:

- Mix the cornflour with a little warm water to make a smooth paste.
- Add the paste to the stock and whisk together well.
- Mix the tomato puree and chopped tomatoes together.
- Place all the ingredients, except the yoghurt and parsley, in the slow cooker.
- Combine gently, season, cover and leave to cook on high for 2-3 hours or until the vegetables are soft and the sauce has thickened.
- Serve in shallow bowls with a dollop of yoghurt sprinkled with chopped parsley.

Ingredients:

2 tsp cornflour
60ml/¼ cup vegetable stock/broth
400g/14oz tinned chopped tomatoes
2 tbsp tomato puree/paste
1kg/2¼lb cauliflower & broccoli florets
½ tsp rock salt
1 onion, sliced
4 tbsp fat free Greek yoghurt
4 tbsp freshly chopped flat leaf parsley
Salt & pepper to taste

If you need to thicken the sauce remove the lid and continue to cook until the sauce reduces down.

Puy Lentils & Sundried Tomatoes
Serves 4

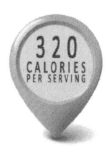

320 CALORIES PER SERVING

Ingredients:

1 tbsp olive oil
250g/9oz puy lentils
150g/5oz courgettes/
zucchini, sliced
150g/5oz green beans,
roughly chopped
75g/3oz sundried
tomatoes, chopped
3 leeks, finely sliced
370ml/1 ½ cups vegetable
stock/broth
250ml/1 cup white wine
4 tbsp soy sauce
Salt & pepper to taste

Method:

• Place all the ingredients in the slow cooker.
• Combine gently, cover and leave to cook on high for 2-3 hours or until the lentils are soft and the stock has been absorbed.
• Season and serve.

You may need to adjust the stock levels and/or cooking time to ensure the lentils are tender and the stock is absorbed.

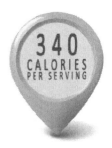

340
CALORIES
PER SERVING

Apricots & Spiced Chickpeas
Serves 4

Method:

• Gently sauté the onions and garlic in a little low cal oil for a few minutes until softened.

• Place all the ingredients, except the chopped coriander & lemon wedges, in the slow cooker.

• Combine gently, season, cover and leave to cook on high for 1-3 hours or until the vegetables are tender.

• Sprinkle with chopped coriander and serve with lemon wedges.

Ingredients:

2 onions, sliced
2 garlic cloves, crushed
400g/14oz tinned chickpeas, rinsed
1 aubergine/eggplant, cubed
150g/5oz courgettes/ zucchini, sliced
75g/3oz dried apricots, chopped
250ml/1 cup tomato passata/sieved tomatoes
1 tsp each ground turmeric, coriander/ cilantro & cumin
½ tsp ground cinnamon
4 tbsp freshly chopped coriander/cilantro
1 lemon, cut into wedges
Low cal cooking oil spray
Salt & pepper to taste

You could use fresh tomatoes and a little vegetable stock rather than passata is you prefer.

Caramelised Ginger Sweet Potatoes
Serves 4

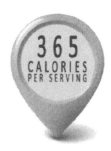

365 CALORIES PER SERVING

Ingredients:

600g/1lb 5oz sweet potatoes, cubed
1 tbsp olive oil
2 tbsp water
2 garlic cloves, crushed
1 onion, sliced
1 tbsp freshly grated ginger
1 tbsp brown sugar
1 tsp each paprika & all spice
Salt & pepper to taste

Method:

• Place all the ingredients in the slow cooker.
• Combine well, season, cover and leave to cook on high for 2-4 hours or until the potatoes are tender.
• Season and serve.

These sweet potatoes are delicious. Make sure they don't 'burn' by stirring and adding a little more water to the slow cooker during cooking if needed.

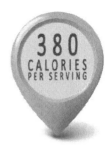

380 CALORIES PER SERVING

Spiced Cauliflower & Veg
Serves 4

Method:

• Place all the ingredients, except the yoghurt, in the slow cooker.

• Combine well, season, cover and leave to cook on high for 2-4 hours or until all the vegetables are tender but still firm.

• Stir through the yoghurt, season and serve.

Ingredients:

1 large cauliflower, broken into florets
200g/7oz potatoes, cubed
200g/7oz green beans, sliced
200g/7oz mushrooms
200g/7oz tinned chickpeas, drained
2 carrots, cut into batons
2 tbsp tomato puree/paste
2 garlic cloves, crushed
1 onion, sliced
½ tsp brown sugar
1 ½ tbsp curry powder
1 tsp paprika
50g/2oz sultanas
250ml/1 cup vegetable stock
3 tbsp fat free Greek yoghurt
Salt & pepper to taste

You could serve the yoghurt on the side with a sprinkle of paprika rather than stirring through the dish.

Mexican Onions
& Kidney Beans
Serves 4

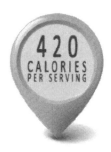

420 CALORIES PER SERVING

Ingredients:

3 large onions, sliced
3 garlic cloves, crushed
1 tbsp olive oil
1 tbsp paprika
1 tsp cumin
1 tbsp sweet chilli sauce
100g/7oz potatoes, chopped
400g/14oz tinned kidney beans, rinsed
200g/7oz mushrooms
3 tbsp tomato puree/paste
250ml/1 cup tomato passata/sieved tomatoes
4 tbsp fat free Greek yoghurt
2 tbsp freshly chopped coriander/cilantro
Salt & pepper to taste

Method:

• Gently sauté the onions and garlic in the olive oil for a few minutes.
• Mix the paprika and cumin with a little warm water to make a paste and stir this through the onions. Continue to cook for a minute or two, add the sweet chilli sauce and combine well.
• Place all the ingredients, except the yoghurt and chopped coriander, in the slow cooker. Stir, season, cover and leave to cook on high for 1-3 hours or until all the vegetables are tender.
• Serve in shallow bowls with a tbsp of yoghurt on the top of each bowl, sprinkled with fresh coriander.

Feel free to spice this dish up further with fresh chopped chillies or ground cayenne pepper.

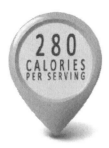

280 CALORIES PER SERVING

Chang Dal
Serves 4

Method:

• Gently sauté the onions and garlic in the olive oil for a few minutes until softened.

• Place all the ingredients, except the yoghurt and chapatti bread, in the slow cooker.

• Stir, season, cover and leave to cook on high for 2-4 hours or until all the chang dal is tender (you may need to add more stock).

• Serve in shallow bowls with yoghurt and chapatti bread on the side.

Ingredients:

2 onions, sliced
3 garlic cloves
1 tbsp olive oil
250g/9oz chang dal
1 tsp each turmeric, coriander/cilantro, cumin & chilli powder
½ tsp garam masala
5 curry leaves
1 tbsp freshly grated ginger
100g/7oz potatoes, chopped
500ml/2 cups vegetable stock/broth
4 tbsp fat free Greek yoghurt
4 regular chapatti breads
Salt & pepper to taste

Chang Dal is an attractive yellow chickpea, which has been stripped of its husk.

Basil 'Pesto' Linguini
Serves 4

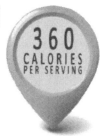

360 CALORIES PER SERVING

Ingredients:

1 handful pine nuts
2 garlic cloves
1 tbsp parmesan cheese
1 tsp rock salt
2 tbsp lemon juice
1 large bunch basil leaves
150g/5oz asparagus tips, roughly chopped
250g/9oz portabella mushrooms, sliced
60ml/ ¼ cup vegetable stock/broth
200g/7oz linguine
2 tbsp low fat crème fraiche
Salt & pepper to taste

Method:

• Add the pine nuts, garlic cloves, parmesan cheese, salt & lemon juice to a food processor and pulse to a fine mixture.
• Place all the ingredients, except the linguine & crème fraiche in the slow cooker. Combine gently, cover and leave to cook on high for 1-2 hours or until the vegetables are tender.
• Meanwhile cook the linguine in salted boiling water until tender.
• Toss the cooked vegetables and linguine together along with the crème fraiche.
• Season well and serve.

This is not a true pesto but it's a lighter olive oil-free alternative. Adjust the salt, lemon and garlic to your own taste.

90

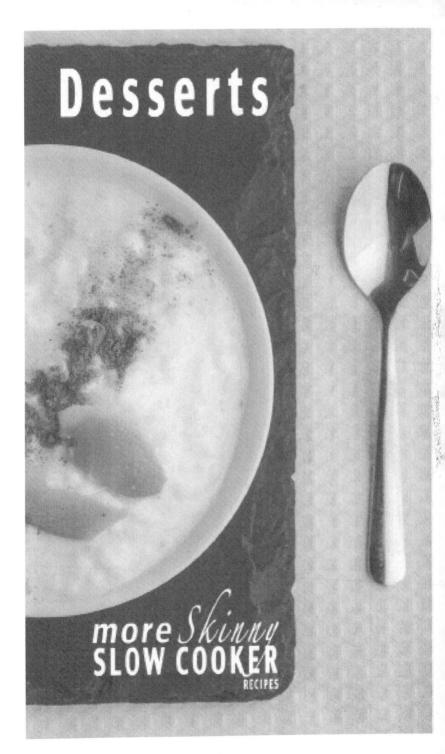

Desserts

more *Skinny*
SLOW COOKER
RECIPES

Fig Stuffed Apples
Serves 4

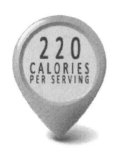

220 CALORIES PER SERVING

Ingredients:

4 Granny Smith cooking apples
200g/7oz dried figs, finely chopped
3 tbsp brown sugar
½ tsp ground cinnamon
60ml/¼ cup apple juice
4 tbsp low fat crème fraiche

Method:

• Core the apples to make a cylindrical hole right through each apple.
• Mix together the chopped figs, sugar and apple juice.
• Stuff each apple with the fig mixture and place in the slow cooker sitting upright.
• Cover and cook for 4-5 hours on low or until the apples are tender.
• Remove the apples, spoon over any juices at the bottom of the slow cooker and serve with a dollop of crème fraiche.

You could use raisins or any other dried fruit you prefer for this recipe.

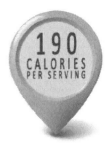

190
CALORIES
PER SERVING

Golden Apricots
Serves 4

Method:

- Take the stones out of the apricots and cut in half.
- Mix together the sugar and apple juice and pour over the top of the apricots in the slow cooker.
- Sprinkle with a little nutmeg.
- Cover and cook for 2-4 hours on low or until the apricots are tender.
- Remove the apricot halves, spoon over any juices at the bottom of the slow cooker and serve with a dollop of yoghurt on top.

Ingredients:

8 ripe apricots
3 tbsp brown sugar
Pinch nutmeg
60ml/¼ cup apple juice
4 tbsp fat free Greek yoghurt

Add a little more apple juice during cooking if you think it needs loosening up.

Nutella Pears
Serves 4

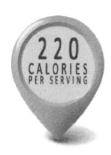

220 CALORIES PER SERVING

Ingredients:

4 ripe pears
3 tbsp nutella
250ml/1 cup apple juice

Method:

• Core the pears and cut them each in half lengthways.

• Gently heat together the nutella and apple juice in a saucepan until warmed and well combined.

• Pour the mixture over the top of the pears in the slow cooker and combine well. Cover and cook for 2-4 hours on low or until the pears are tender.

• Remove the pear halves and spoon over the chocolate & apple sauce.

A little single cream or milk is a lovely addition to this dish but it will increase the calories, so don't over-do it.

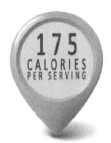

Vanilla & Bananas

Serves 4

Method:

- Peel the bananas and slice in half lengthways.
- Gently heat together the sugar and pineapple juice in a saucepan until the sugar has dissolved to make a syrup.
- Add the vanilla essence and pour the vanilla syrup over the top of the bananas in the slow cooker. Cover and cook for 1-2 hours on low.
- Remove the bananas and spoon the syrup over the top with a dollop of Greek yoghurt.

Ingredients:

4 bananas
1 tsp vanilla extract
3 tbsp brown sugar
120ml/½ cup pineapple juice
4 tbsp fat free Greek yoghurt

Crème fraiche will work just as well for this recipe.

Rice Pudding
Serves 4

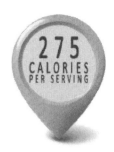

275
CALORIES
PER SERVING

Ingredients:

200g/7oz Arborio rice
500ml/2 cups skimmed milk
2 tbsp runny honey
1 free range egg, beaten
½ tsp cinnamon

Method:

• Add all the ingredients to the slow cooker.
• Combine well, cover and leave to cook on high for 2-3 hours or until the rice pudding is tender.

Keep an eye on the texture during cooking; add a little more milk if needed or increase the cooking time to thicken the pudding up.

CONVERSION CHART: DRY INGREDIENTS

Metric	Imperial
7g	¼ oz
15g	½ oz
20g	¾ oz
25g	1 oz
40g	1½oz
50g	2oz
60g	2½oz
75g	3oz
100g	3½oz
125g	4oz
140g	4½oz
150g	5oz
165g	5½oz
175g	6oz
200g	7oz
225g	8oz
250g	9oz
275g	10oz
300g	11oz
350g	12oz
375g	13oz
400g	14oz

Metric	Imperial
425g	15oz
450g	1lb
500g	1lb 2oz
550g	1¼lb
600g	1lb 5oz
650g	1lb 7oz
675g	1½lb
700g	1lb 9oz
750g	1lb 11oz
800g	1¾lb
900g	2lb
1kg	2¼lb
1.1kg	2½lb
1.25kg	2¾lb
1.35kg	3lb
1.5kg	3lb 6oz
1.8kg	4lb
2kg	4½lb
2.25kg	5lb
2.5kg	5½lb
2.75kg	6lb

CONVERSION CHART: LIQUID MEASURES

Metric	Imperial	US
25ml	1fl oz	
60ml	2fl oz	¼ cup
75ml	2½ fl oz	
100ml	3½fl oz	
120ml	4fl oz	½ cup
150ml	5fl oz	
175ml	6fl oz	
200ml	7fl oz	
250ml	8½ fl oz	1 cup
300ml	10½ fl oz	
360ml	12½ fl oz	
400ml	14fl oz	
450ml	15½ fl oz	
600ml	1 pint	
750ml	1¼ pint	3 cups
1 litre	1½ pints	4 cups

Other
COOKNATION
TITLES

If you enjoyed 'More Skinny Slow Cooker Recipes' we'd really appreciate your feedback. Reviews help others decide if this is the right book for them so a moment of your time would be appreciated.

Thank you.

You may also be interested in other '**Skinny**' titles in the CookNation series. You can find all the following great titles by searching under '**CookNation**'.

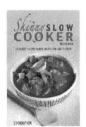

The Skinny Slow Cooker Recipe Book

Delicious Recipes Under 300, 400 And 500 Calories.

Paperback / eBook

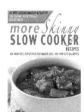

More Skinny Slow Cooker Recipes

75 More Delicious Recipes Under 300, 400 & 500 Calories.

Paperback / eBook

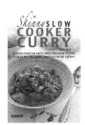

The Skinny Slow Cooker Curry Recipe Book

Low Calorie Curries From Around The World

Paperback / eBook

The Skinny Slow Cooker Soup Recipe Book

Simple, Healthy & Delicious Low Calorie Soup Recipes For Your Slow Cooker. All Under 100, 200 & 300 Calories.

Paperback / eBook

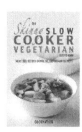

The Skinny Slow Cooker Vegetarian Recipe Book

40 Delicious Recipes Under 200, 300 And 400 Calories.

Paperback / eBook

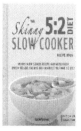

The Skinny 5:2 Slow Cooker Recipe Book

Skinny Slow Cooker Recipe And Menu Ideas Under 100, 200, 300 & 400 Calories For Your 5:2 Diet.

Paperback / eBook

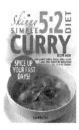

The Skinny 5:2 Curry Recipe Book

Spice Up Your Fast Days With Simple Low Calorie Curries, Snacks, Soups, Salads & Sides Under 200, 300 & 400 Calories

Paperback / eBook

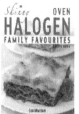

The Skinny Halogen Oven Family Favourites Recipe Book

Healthy, Low Calorie Family Meal-Time Halogen Oven Recipes Under 300, 400 and 500 Calories

Paperback / eBook

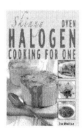

Skinny Halogen Oven Cooking For One

Single Serving, Healthy, Low Calorie Halogen Oven Recipes Under 200, 300 and 400 Calories

Paperback / eBook

Skinny Winter Warmers Recipe Book

Soups, Stews, Casseroles & One Pot Meals Under 300, 400 & 500 Calories.

Paperback / eBook

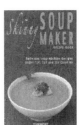

The Skinny Soup Maker Recipe Book

Delicious Low Calorie, Healthy and Simple Soup Recipes Under 100, 200 and 300 Calories. Perfect For Any Diet and Weight Loss Plan.

Paperback / eBook

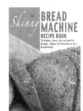

The Skinny Bread Machine Recipe Book

70 Simple, Lower Calorie, Healthy Breads...Baked To Perfection In Your Bread Maker.

Paperback / eBook

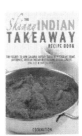

The Skinny Indian Takeaway Recipe Book

Authentic British Indian Restaurant Dishes Under 300, 400 And 500 Calories. The Secret To Low Calorie Indian Takeaway Food At Home

Paperback / eBook

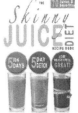

The Skinny Juice Diet Recipe Book

5lbs, 5 Days. The Ultimate Kick-Start Diet and Detox Plan to Lose Weight & Feel Great!

Paperback / eBook

Available only on eBook

The Skinny 5:2 Diet Recipe Book Collection

All The 5:2 Fast Diet Recipes You'll Ever Need. All Under 100, 200, 300, 400 And 500 Calories

eBook

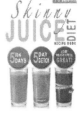

The Skinny 5:2 Fast Diet Meals For One

Single Serving Fast Day Recipes & Snacks Under 100, 200 & 300 Calories

Paperback / eBook

The Skinny 5:2 Fast Diet Vegetarian Meals For One

Single Serving Fast Day Recipes & Snacks Under 100, 200 & 300 Calories

Paperback / eBook

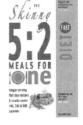

The Skinny 5:2 Fast Diet Family Favourites Recipe Book

Eat With All The Family On Your Diet Fasting Days

Paperback / eBook

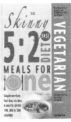

Available only on eBook

The Skinny 5:2 Fast Diet Family Favorites Recipe Book *U.S.A. EDITION*

Dine With All The Family On Your Diet Fasting Days

Paperback / eBook

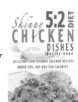

The Skinny 5:2 Diet Chicken Dishes Recipe Book

Delicious Low Calorie Chicken Dishes Under 300, 400 & 500 Calories

Paperback / eBook

103

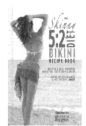

The Skinny 5:2 Bikini Diet Recipe Book

Recipes & Meal Planners Under 100, 200 & 300 Calories. Get Ready For Summer & Lose Weight...FAST!

Paperback / eBook

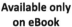

The Paleo Diet For Beginners Slow Cooker Recipe Book

Gluten Free, Everyday Essential Slow Cooker Paleo Recipes For Beginners

Available only on eBook

eBook

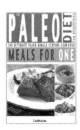

The Paleo Diet For Beginners Meals For One

The Ultimate Paleo Single Serving Cookbook

Paperback / eBook

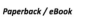

The Paleo Diet For Beginners Holidays

Thanksgiving, Christmas & New Year Paleo Friendly Recipes

Available only on eBook

eBook

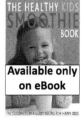

Available only on eBook

The Healthy Kids Smoothie Book

40 Delicious Goodness In A Glass Recipes for Happy Kids.

eBook

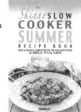

The Skinny Slow Cooker Summer Recipe Book

Fresh & Seasonal Summer Recipes For Your Slow Cooker. All Under 300, 400 And 500 Calories.

Paperback / eBook

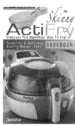
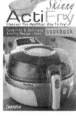

The Skinny ActiFry Cookbook

Guilt-free and Delicious ActiFry Recipe Ideas: Discover The Healthier Way to Fry!

Paperback / eBook

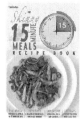

The Skinny 15 Minute Meals Recipe Book

Delicious, Nutritious & Super-Fast Meals in 15 Minutes Or Less. All Under 300, 400 & 500 Calories.

Paperback / eBook

The Skinny Mediterranean Recipe Book

Simple, Healthy & Delicious Low Calorie Mediterranean Diet Dishes. All Under 200, 300 & 400 Calories.

Paperback / eBook

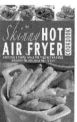

The Skinny Hot Air Fryer Cookbook

Delicious & Simple Meals For Your Hot Air Fryer: Discover The Healthier Way To Fry.

Paperback / eBook

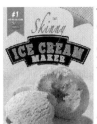

The Skinny Ice Cream Maker

Delicious Lower Fat, Lower Calorie Ice Cream, Frozen Yogurt & Sorbet Recipes For Your Ice Cream Maker

Paperback / eBook

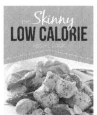

The Skinny Low Calorie Recipe Book

Great Tasting, Simple & Healthy Meals Under 300, 400 & 500 Calories. Perfect For Any Calorie Controlled Diet.

Paperback / eBook

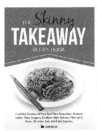

The Skinny Takeaway Recipe Book

Healthier Versions Of Your Fast Food Favourites: Chinese, Indian, Pizza, Burgers, Southern Style Chicken, Mexican & More. All Under 300, 400 & 500 Calories

Paperback / eBook

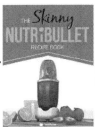

The Skinny Nutribullet Recipe Book

80+ Delicious & Nutritious Healthy Smoothie Recipes. Burn Fat, Lose Weight and Feel Great!

Paperback / eBook

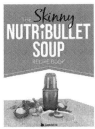

The Skinny Nutribullet Soup Recipe Book

Delicious, Quick & Easy, Single Serving Soups & Pasta Sauces For Your Nutribullet. All Under 100, 200, 300 & 400 Calories.

Paperback / eBook

19824829R00060

Printed in Great Britain
by Amazon